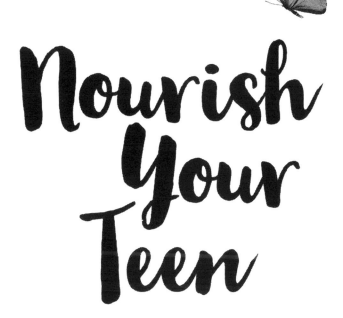

# Nourish Your Teen

## mind, body and soul

### A practical toolkit

# KELLY ROSE

## RNutr

ISBN 978-1-912145-74-4

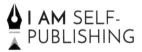 I AM SELF-
PUBLISHING

# Contents

# Preface

It was a sunny Easter Sunday morning as I jogged through the village with Toby, our little wire-haired Fox Terrier. The morning was cool and I noticed the beautiful daffodils were out in force, contrasting with the green grass which always makes me feel super alive, free and connected to everything. I surrendered to the divine and asked for a miracle. I had known for some time I wanted to write a book and had started at least four different titles, but each time the ego self had seemed to step in and tell me that I wasn't ready or good enough. Today felt different; I was ready. I had been listening to Marianne Williamson's A Return to Love workshop and so I offered up my confusion, chaos and tendency to overwork up to the divine and felt myself let go, as she suggested. I asked, "What will you have me do?' Which book should I write? I want to help others, so what is the message I can give? Please tell me what you want me to write?"

My heart was open and I felt my bliss. As I passed my village church, the lady vicar crossed the road and came directly in my path. I do not think of myself as a particularly religious person and like so many of us, attend church only for special occasions, such as Christmas, weddings, christenings and funerals. I had been listening to the inspiring Marianne Williamson telling her audience about there being no accidents and chance encounters, and here was the lady vicar greeting me, and I her. It was a very brief meeting, but it meant much more to me. It was a sign that the universe 'had my back' – I was ready.

I returned home and as I busied myself in the kitchen, an idea popped into my mind and I knew this was it: 'Nourish your teen's mind, body and soul.' At that moment, everything came flooding in. I had been preparing to write this book all of my life; in fact, I had always been leading up to this. After all, my own teenage years had included some of the darkest and most painful times in my life. I teach teenagers and I am lucky to have two beautiful daughters, one of whom is a teen and the other swiftly approaching that age. As a young girl, I felt confused and became obsessed with inwardly asking myself: 'Why am I here?' and 'What is the purpose of my life?' Through writing this book and following my own path, I now understand that these questions are normal for a young girl going through a time of great change.

Every single one of us has a part to play in this life, even if we don't want to acknowledge it or are unable to do so. I feel gratitude every day for receiving the gift of being a guide to these two special and unique beings. I fully believe that each of us is important and so no one else can take your place in this life. You are supposed to be here and you are simply love. Fear is a mere illusion and it is our job to work through our fears to get to the joyful moments.

# Introduction

Being a parent to teens is, to say the least, a challenge. While the baby, infant and child stages come with numerous demands of their own, I feel these have been quite extensively written about and can be navigated a tad more easily than the teenage stage. Maybe this is because we start to sense both our child's growing independence and our own freedom as we no longer need to keep them occupied, fed, dry, hydrated and dressed. Then, bang! The mood swings arrive, the emotional testing, the worry that our teen is making poor decisions, and more! Maybe it's because we feel aggrieved by this irritable, untidy being who has replaced our sweet smiley baby, which leaves us with the overwhelming we have lost parental control. Whatever the issues, I can tell you there is no going back.

One of the reasons I started to write this book was that I kept hearing the older generation around us make statements like: "When your children are young, it is the best times of your life." This was accompanied by a shake of the head and an expression that told you the best times were behind you and you just had to move forward to teen parenthood with dread. I decided this was not the mindset for me and I would never repeat this when I became a parent of 'older children'. It just needs a shift in perception. There is a challenge at every age for a parent, so I implore you to read through this book, communicate with your child, continue to learn from them and keep growing as a parent. If you do, you will find joy at every opportunity.

If I had only one aim for this book, it would be to enable children to overcome challenges, realise they can be repaired and understand that life is a cycle of ups and downs. Every person experiences this cycle in a myriad of ways, the only difference is how we react and move through each of the highs and lows. As a teacher, I see students react in many different ways and I also see both of my children reacting to situations in a way that is unique to their personalities and needs.

One fifth of our adolescents could experience a mental health problem within the space of one year[1]. Many people suggest that anxiety and mental illness is on the increase and it is disturbing, as a parent, to note that 50 per cent of mental health issues are established by the age of 14[2]. It really makes you think about what we can do to set our children up to thrive in the present world. With a few simple shifts in our thinking, I believe we can guide the future generation to a life of happiness and appreciation.

Viktor Frankl is the author of one of the most remarkable books I have ever read, Man's Search for Meaning. He tells of his plight in surviving the holocaust and gives an in-depth account of his experiences in the concentration camps. It may seem extreme to mention this in a book about teens of the 21st century, but I believe we can learn a lot from Frankl's writings while tackling present day issues. I have obtained a deep sense of how powerful the human mind really is from his writings, and how each person must find meaning, no

---

[1] WHO (2003), Caring for Children and Adolescents with Mental Disorders: Setting WHO Directions. [online] Geneva: World Health Organization. Available at: http://www.who.int/mental_health/media/en/785.pdf (3 July 2016)

[2] https://www.mentalhealth.org.uk/statistics/mental-health-statistics-children-and-young-people

matter what the circumstances of their life are. If your child can understand they are valuable and matter, this will create an essential foundation to their life.

It is part of my role in a secondary school to incorporate lessons, programmes, events, strategies and interventions to support the development of emotional resilience and positive mental health. We each have a brain; therefore, we each have a level of mental health. This is important for us all to remember. Just as your body must be cared for in order to thrive, so must your mind. It took me a while to grasp this concept as we tend to think of exercising our body as a norm and ignore the mind. Exercise for the mind supports inner joy and peace, as well as strengthening our willpower and self-control, which improves our decision-making processes. It also encourages greater focus and self-awareness, the keys to a successful and happy life.

Many children in our society carry a heavy weight of emotional baggage from their early relationships. Attachment issues are on the increase, which has resulted in poor behavioural self-control becoming more prevalent in the classroom. These young people want to be listened to and need to have strong positive role models in their lives. They each deserve to be able to contribute to our society as a valuable citizen. I entered the teaching profession later than most and was surprised to find – I suppose naively – that the most humbling part of the role is that every day a teacher makes a difference, and that is not purely centred around the teaching of a subject. This is even more powerful if you are a parent or guardian, as just the way that you greet your child each morning can affect the way they see themselves.

Every part of this book is a guide to emotional resilience, not just for our children, but also for us – as parents, aunties, uncles, friends, educators and responsible citizens. A positive and strong level of mental health can be achieved by building on the habits, thought processes and strategies within these pages. So take your time, make notes and reread the parts that resonate with you. Enjoy your journey, as being a children's guide provides a wonderful reason for being here on this Earth and living out this one amazing life that we have!

I hope, as you read through this book, it will cradle and support you through the hardest times of being a parent or guide and continue to be a reference in many situations. After all, guiding children is an amazing gift; it is also abundant, with unforeseeable challenges and lessons that call for our very best selves.

Forgive the educator in me, but the following are a few rules that will support your parental mindset and help you to guide your teen. The first is to engage with the following concept; you are a parent and not a friend to your teen (although you can be both eventually). You have to be prepared to be not liked and even hated occasionally, it really is a part of the job. It is part of the process, perhaps the hardest, and completely usual. The second is to develop a self-care practice for yourself. Your well-being is essential if you are to become the parent you desire to be. I once had the notion that I was to be a martyr and would give every part of me, 150 per cent, to being a parent, so that my daughters could be happy – crazy! Now I realise, from my own personal experience, that children will only thrive when you are happy and healthy. Therefore, leave the 'me time' guilt behind, it will benefit your whole family.

> Health is a state of complete physical, mental and social well-being and not merely the absence of disease or infirmity.  WHO

# Chapter 1

# The three Cs

The underlying principles throughout this book are incorporated into three Cs - contact, consistency and communication. If you take nothing more from this book, thinking about and implement the three C will change your relationship with your teen for the better.

1. **Contact**
   Demonstrate that you love your child with regular hugs, smiles, encouraging words or gentle head strokes. There will be times when they are unwelcome, so do not ever force it, but do gently reassure them that your love is unconditional. We all want to be secure in the knowledge that we are loved, even when we are displaying behaviours that are driven by hormones, brain changes and things beyond our control. Knowing that you are loved, no matter what, gives you great power and a feeling of worthiness. My oldest daughter is not always receptive to hugs and it can at times be easier to let her be; however, I know that it is even more important to assure her that she is loved at these times.

2. **Consistency**
   Always follow through with promises and discipline. Your teen needs to know that you love them enough to keep your word and enforce boundaries. In fact, contrary to what you may think, shaky boundaries and inconsistency can lead to great confusion and low self-esteem. Every

young person needs to know there are rules they must keep and values to uphold. This helps them to feel safe and develops their confidence. Remember, you are being observed constantly, so it is important to try and practice what you preach. I want to stress, however, that we are all conditioned by our own past. Therefore, the 'perfect' parent does not exist. (See Embrace your imperfection, below, for more on this subject.) Should you make a mistake or act in the wrong way, forgive yourself and take note of the third C.

3. **Communication**

Be interested in your teen's life, even when they enter secondary school stage and become a little secretive. Bear with it, avoid direct questions and keep up to date with their friends, teachers and lessons, and support them in their hobbies or activities. Welcome their friends into your home and make your home a sanctuary and safe place for them to be upset without feeling judged. Engage in one-to-one conversations and arrange together time. When your child knows you are really listening, they will want to share more with you and their self-esteem will develop naturally. A good tip here is to keep mealtimes a no technology zone and that goes for all of the family. Setting some rules helps communication rather than hinders it, and setting family rules together opens up communication even further.

## Embrace your imperfection

I am an imperfect parent and invite you to be an imperfect parent too. When we let go of the idea that we have to be everything to everyone and work ourselves into the ground doing so, we can really get to grips with being a great parent. I read so many books on parenting because I wanted to make

sure my children were confident, happy, educated, polite…
and the list goes on. However, as a result of teaching young
people and parenting my own children, I can tell you that if
you want to ensure your child is all of those things, you have
to work on being these things yourself. When I say 'work', I
mean invest time in your own personal growth and self-love.
You are amazing and deserve to feel so.

Marianne Williams  You are
imperfect until
you are not.

Life is a journey and we learn and heal throughout. This
means there will always be ups and downs, spikes and
troughs throughout our lives. The best thing you can do is to
be yourself with your child and show them that we all make
mistakes and learn from them. I labour this point because I
want you to know that even as I write this book, to inspire
you and support your love for both yourself and your teen,
I also understand that I have so much more to learn and
there is always more to know. I make mistakes daily and
confess this with the hope that you will feel free to be you,
and will use the three Cs to gain strength for your parental
journey. You will be a better parent when you embrace your
imperfections and let go of being 'perfect'.

How do you react when you make a mistake? Do you beat
yourself up verbally, do you call yourself names and become
annoyed, even angry? Forgiving yourself is the first step and
then by incorporating rule number 6, you can really support
healthy family relationships.

## Rule number 6

I first read the story of rule number 6 in James Altucher's book, The Power of No, and then saw it again in The Art of Possibility by Rosamund and Ben Zander. It made me giggle each time I told it to friends, the young people I teach and my own family. It became a lovely shared joke that lightened the mood and lived out its purpose every time. Here is the story of rule number 6 for you; I hope it can serve you in the same way.

Two Prime Ministers were sitting in a room when suddenly the door burst open and a man entered extremely upset, shouting and gesticulating wildly. The resident Prime Minister said gently, "Peter, Peter, please remember rule number 6." Almost immediately the gentleman was restored to complete calm.

After a time a young woman came in. She was hysterical, her hair and arms flying all over the place. The home country Prime Minister calmly said, "Maria, please remember rule number 6," and again Maria bowed, apologised profusely, and respectfully left the room.

After a third time, the visiting Prime Minister was extremely curious and asked, "My dear colleague, I've seen three people come into the room in a state of uncontrollable fury and walk out completely calmly. Would you be willing to share what rule number 6 is?"

The resident Prime Minister responded, "Oh, yes, rule number 6 is very simple. Don't take yourself so damned seriously."

The visiting Prime Minister said: "Oh, that's a wonderful rule. What, may I ask, are the other rules?"

The resident Prime Minister replied: "There aren't any."

**LINKS**

http://www.creatingthe21stcentury.org/Katalina3-Rule6.html

There you have it - life is just a story that we tell ourselves. When we get mad and tied up in our own pride, needs and wants, rule number 6 can come in and remind us to not take it all so seriously and laugh instead. Laughing is a medicine when we get caught in the ego mind.

Ryan Holiday
*Ego is the Enemy*

**Those who have subdued their ego understand that it doesn't degrade you when others treat you poorly; it degrades them.**

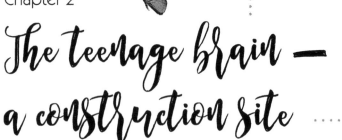

# Chapter 2

# The teenage brain — a construction site

Part way through the writing of this book, I came across the most wonderful resource in the form of the book, Your Teenager is Not Crazy by Dr Jeramy Clark and his wife, Jerusha Clark. I related so much to the theory and the clever analogy of a construction site they use to explain up-to-date science on the teenage brain. The creative couple write that 'teenagers are not crazy', they are just undergoing 'an amazing period of neurological opportunity'. You will find this book invaluable if you are bringing up a teen, as it provides an in-depth understanding of your child's brain and explains why they may seem to have changed completely overnight. I wanted to share this with you here to help you to understand that the change you see in your teen is completely normal and embracing this period of time will only help you and your teen to flourish.

If, like me, you have felt resistance in the not so distant past as you tried to grip tightly to that sweet little child that once was, please don't despair; they are coming back and they do still need you. As the couple so perceptibly implore their readers in the book, you must 'don your construction hat' and 'stay on site', as 'connection' could well be an additional C in this book. My own teenage years have left me with a heightened awareness and instinct that keeping yourself connected with your teens by being supportive and non-judgemental during and after this period will ensure that the parts of their personality you love will shine through and come back. However, I must also stress it is important to be extremely mindful that we are purely guides, these young people do not belong to us. Therefore, keeping boundaries and exploring all of the topics described in this book will ensure they continue to thrive and learn during their unique journeys. It can be a tricky balancing act on a tightrope!

'I'm bored.' This dreaded statement makes even the most patient of parents bristle, as the idea of being bored is a mere luxury for us and the tendency to lecture is so powerful. It may surprise you (it did me) that being uncomfortable, stressed or having the urge to relieve boredom is essential to the development of your teen. Allowing your child to feel bored and find their own way is crucial, so try to resist the urge to berate them with a long list of jobs, which was my go-to strategy. Instead, try to empathise and focus on doing new things with your teens when you are able to. So try being adventurous with some new foods and making it a fun activity, or have fun trying a new sport or task. Whatever you do, try and direct this normal period of boredom towards positive experiences, avoiding leaving them alone to partake in risk-taking behaviour. Your task is to find out what gets your teen interested and excited, rather than doing the same things you always have done, and you may find something new that you absolutely love too. My children love to cook, experiment in the kitchen, dance and be out in nature, which is good for me too. Occasionally, participating in a new activity with your teen will promote the adventurous and independent side of your child in a positive way.

Not all teenagers react to this brain reconstruction phase in the same way and scientists suggest there may be links to these changes in the brain with a teenager's conflicting extremes in attitude. Around the age of 11, the brain starts to grow at speed; it can be likened to a tree branching off and making more connections, followed by a pruning process. This is the construction stage already mentioned. During this pruning process, scientists suggest that certain parts of the brain become less responsive. This is relevant to you as a parent because tests show that teenagers find facial expressions extremely difficult to read. Has your teen ever made a snap judgement before you've even had time to open your mouth that was completely off course and contrary to what you were actually thinking? Has your teen misread your intentions because of this brain upheaval? It certainly makes you think, doesn't it? It also makes the communication process and finding the time to communicate all the more important. If you would like to find out more about these changes in the brain, Nicola Morgan explains the full science in an interesting way that is easy to understand in her book Blame my Brain. It is written for teens, but is also a fantastic resource for us guides.

References: *Your Teenager is Not Crazy* by Dr Jeramy Clark and Jerusha Clark, and *Blame my Brain* by Nicola Morgan.

Chapter 3

# Actions speak louder than your words and your truth is precious

You can tell your child they are beautiful morning, noon and night, but if you do not feel it within yourself they will pick up on this, no matter how strong your words are. Your children watch you and we know that learned behaviour is a common phenomenon. For example, if you tell your children not to lie and then lie yourself about a parental break-up, fight, disagreement or something else, in a well meaning, purely protective way. When possible, be honest with your child, as secrets and lies can build resentment and create distance in families. Your child is more resilient than you think and being honest and supportive will encourage their growth in a positive way.

Albert Schweitzer

> Example is not the main thing in influencing others, it is the only thing.

There will be situations when your children are too young to interpret or understand certain information and, of course, here you must give them time to grow up. However, in most cases, my advice is to give an honest and appropriate answer. Your teens will respect you for being truthful and take your lead in being respectful and avoid lying to you. Note: lies breed deception.

Demonstrate what it means to make choices and be firm when your teen seems to make an inappropriate choice (expect this, it is part of the process) and provide a consequence, if it's required. You should also reinforce the appropriate action or choice and use real-life situations or stories to help them understand the possible outcomes of making different decisions. This is important because your teen can find it extremely challenging to not act impulsively and use rational reasoning. To help you here, keep in mind that your teen is very receptive to rewards. Therefore, knowing what gets them motivated is essential in keeping them directed towards a positive path. Rewards should be individual to your child, so listen to them and learn; examples could be money to buy clothes, materials for a hobby, time to play a computer game or watch a film, or being out with their friends. As mentioned earlier, it would be more unusual if your teen did not make mistakes. After all, mistakes are merely learning opportunities, not just for them, but also for parents. I confess to making snap judgements and I apologise when I make them. I am human, after all. If we can aim to be patient and try to understand why our teen has made a particular choice, we can help them to choose differently next time. The following statements may help you next time you are about to fly off the handle in disbelief at a seemingly crazy situation (oh, and you may need to take a deep breath first).

*"Please tell me why you... It is just that I would like to understand."*

*"I know you wouldn't mean to cause this… I would like to help us both to understand and maybe I can help you put this right."*

*"I love you unconditionally and mistakes are part of life, we all make them. It is important that we can discuss and learn from them."*

As I said earlier, always show the way, keep communication open, apologise if you make a mistake and show your child how we can put things right. The ego mind - or your 'chimp', as Professor Steven Peters calls it in his book, The Chimp Paradox - does not like to admit being wrong, but would you rather be right or happy? It is amazing how saying you are sorry and explaining yourself moves a situation onto more positive ground.

There have been more than a few times where I have overreacted and, quick as a flash, turned into a raging banshee, allowing my own fear and ego to take over. Beating yourself up mentally is generally the first port of call, isn't it? I remember pouring out my guilt at one of these times to a friend. Then, all of a sudden, I realised that by apologising to my teen and explaining that I had judged them and reacted according to my ego thoughts, I had opened up the lines of communication to my daughter. This led to an open conversation about how I could have dealt with things in a better way, which seemed to repair the relationship and make it stronger than before. I really believe this is because it is good for your child to see you as imperfect. Embracing our imperfections and releasing the need to be right and defensive serves us and our children in a much better way. I have made a commitment to continue to increase my awareness and practice defencelessness, but it is not always easy.

## Would you rather be right or happy?

 WHO

My youngest child is a natural lover of words and, as I write this book, she is a big fan of saying "hypocrite". Once she is given a directive, she takes the role of the rule police and checks to see if the person who is issuing the advice also follows it. She once demonstratively announced that the young man setting out some trampolining safety guidance was 'a hypocrite' as he was wearing shoes whilst instructing them not to. You can see why I am learning to tread carefully with the literacy rule police about…

Here, I remind you again to embrace your imperfection. We are all unique and have our own learned and conditioned behaviours to contend with. Remember that communicating with your teen and being authentically honest will support you in your quest to bring forth the development of a loving, authentic person.

# Chapter 4

# Inspiring your teen to develop resilience

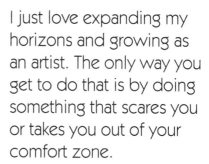

Vanessa Hudgens

> I just love expanding my horizons and growing as an artist. The only way you get to do that is by doing something that scares you or takes you out of your comfort zone.

As parents, we are no strangers to the demands of life and understand that to be successful, have freedom and enjoy life, one must develop resilience and an ability to overcome hardships. I once heard the story of two twins. One fell into the throes of drug addiction and stated that she had 'no choice' because she had been abused as a young child. The other twin was successful in many areas of life and stated that she had 'no choice' because she had been abused as a child. Isn't it fascinating how each person deals with a situation differently?

Getting out of your comfort zone is a must if you want to move forward to experience more happiness, and any resistance to moving on will inevitably push you into some other type of chaos or unhappiness. When I was in my thirties, I discovered that every time I pushed out of my current situation, either by studying, work development or setting myself a challenge, I developed more confidence and belief in myself. I got it! How wonderful to encourage this in our children, to help them understand that it is OK to be nervous, anxious and scared, and that it certainly will not stop them going ahead and reaping the bonus reward at the end of their endeavour.

As an educator, I see many young people rising to challenges. Some switch off from school through fear or because of a specific challenge and some crumble, becoming vulnerable to unhealthy or high risk-taking behaviours. There are even those who you think are performing well and then discover are a ticking time bomb waiting to explode from exam pressure or life in general. Every chapter in this book is focused on developing resilience and encouraging the growth of self-love and confidence by praising positive behaviours and accomplishment, and supporting all of these with mindfulness, gratitude and nourishment. However, by adding the extra encouragement of allowing your child to step out of their comfort zone will equip them with a belief that will help them to soar. Please let me reassure you, I am definitely not talking about releasing them into the wild or placing them, unprepared, into a dangerous or risky situation.

There are many examples I could use, but I will keep it simple. My daughter came to me really upset one day last year; after desperately wanting a part in a school play, she had been given just that. Well, as you can imagine, I was very confused to see her tears. However, the fear that she was feeling at the realisation of having to actually stand up and play the part had overtaken her. She begged me to ask the school to change the part for her and I refused. There were tantrums and more tears. How do you think she felt when she played her part and received wonderful feedback? Exactly! Giving in to our fears is not an option. I remember being scared of going through with my dance exams as a teen. I asked my mum if I could leave the class and that was that, I never went back. I never had the chance to continue with doing something I enjoyed. This is a perfect example of how the illusion of fear can scupper things.

Part of developing a sense of repair and resilience is being able to cope with the natural ups and downs that occur in our lives. At a recent mental health conference (Schools NorthEast Prince Bishops Teaching School Alliance, Newcastle United football ground, Wednesday, 22 June 2016) the figures were startling, as we heard that one in five children will experience mental health problems. It is important for our children to know that our brains need to be cared for as much as our bodies. We all have a level of mental health and we will support learning and happiness by keeping ourselves as healthy and positive as we can.

One of the most concerning behaviours that is on the increase in schools is self-harming, and one of the reasons that young people continue to hurt themselves intentionally is thought to be connected to the rush of endorphins that are released to relieve the pain, which results in a rush of good feelings. It begs the question, "Why do our teens need to harm themselves to feel good?"

How much time does any of us spend doing something that is not connected to any particular outcome, expectation, assessment or purpose? Would self-harming exist if people were to spend 30 minutes every day doing something just for the joy of it? I am aware, as I say this, that many teens would argue they have fun on social media. However, this is not what I am alluding to, as users of these apps and social media sites have many expectations and can confer judgement. Therefore, this is not the 30 minutes of mindfulness that can support positive mental health.

Encourage your teen to do something every day that they enjoy. If it is art therapy, there are many beautiful colouring books out now for all ages. It may be playing a musical instrument or singing just for fun, without the need to prepare for an exam. My girls and I love to put the music on loud and dance around the kitchen. Although this doesn't happen every day, I encourage them to find something that helps them to feel good. This is different for each of them. Ava loves writing, reading, singing and dancing, whilst Abigail enjoys singing, applying makeup, cooking and being active outdoors.

But be aware that even fun exercise can turn into something that you measure. For example, the park run is a wonderful community event that is a major success in the UK, with most part people going along and encouraging each other to be active together. However, be aware of your teen becoming obsessed with timings, as this turns something that should be enjoyable into a pressurised exercise, which is the opposite of mindful.

A few years ago, I wore a bracelet that recorded my timings and calculated my calories as I ran through my village, but quite soon I stopped using it, as I was beginning to obsess about beating my own time, forgetting about the beautiful flowers and the scenic river, which never fails to calm my mind. (This not always a bad thing, as improving yourself is a good mindset to cultivate. However, this was my time to forget about self-improvement and feel gratitude.)

Your child is watching you, so are you taking time out for yourself? Are you looking after your own mental health? Although I have focused on encouraging your teen, it is worth mentioning that they will develop what is 'the norm' from their parents.

## LINKS

http://www.livescience.com/11043-teens-hurt-science-injury.html

Neale Donald Walsch

> Life beings at the end of your comfort zone.

> Courage is not something that you already have... Courage is what you earn when you've been through the tough times and you discover they aren't so tough after all.

Malcolm Gladwell
David and Goliath

27

## Chapter 5

# Feeding the mind of your teen

Encouraging your child to read from an early age is a preferred strategy. Reading and looking at picture books with them when they are young provides them with a grounding and a love of books, and I believe wholeheartedly this has instilled a thirst for learning in both of my girls, albeit in different ways. Please do not despair or feel any guilt if reading has not been part of your child's experience so far, as my own love of books started when I was a teen, as a result of a friend's influence. However, the experience for my first child was not so easy. She loves books but reading at bedtime, which has always been a ritual in our house, became a source of frustration as she first began to learn to read independently.

My eldest daughter has wonderful dyslexic tendencies. I love to frame this in such a way that dyslexia is not who she is. It is merely an extra, and a positive addition at that. After all, Keira Knightley, Richard Branson and numerous other talented, successful beings have also been blessed with dyslexia. One view is that the difficulties and academic failures that a person with dyslexic tendencies experience can lead to an accumulation of strategies to navigate life in a more resilient way. Being educated about specific learning difficulties (SpLD), both independently and within a Master's module, has taught me so much, including how to be a better teacher. It has given me the understanding that we all learn in different ways. Although I could take issue with the word 'difficulties' within SpLD, I agree that it is true in the sense that traditional learning methods do make life difficult for those with dyslexic tendencies.

I will make some suggestions within the nutrition section of this book, but I will otherwise refrain from giving you further insights into the fabulous world of dyslexia because of the book by Dr Eide, The Dyslexia Advantage, says it all so well. Suffice to say, in the early days of her education we were a bit flummoxed as to why she found reading and spelling such a challenge, although seeing me read and the enjoyment of reading books together were instrumental in fostering her natural love of books.

We live in a wonderful age of technology, but you could also argue that there are plenty of negatives as well. However, I will focus here on using technology in our favour. If we do this and utilise all of the strategies that instil a strong sense of self-esteem and self-respect in our teens, we will find the negatives are less of an issue.

The reason I mention technology at this point is that our youths have audiobooks and super sparkling bloggers and vloggers that make it easy for them to gain a positive perspective on life. You may have to do some homework here and help steer viewing in a specific direction. I think it is now futile to try to keep our teens away from technology, but we can certainly have an input into what they are watching or listening to. An informative resource I would recommend on this topic is Sex, Likes and Social Media, a book by Allison Havey and Deana Puccio. Our generation has a very different view on technology and this will open your eyes to the dangers of social media and equip you with the knowledge to allow you to communicate effectively with your adolescent. You could say I have been lucky here, as my children have not once asked to go on Facebook and they have a very good handle on privacy in their accounts. Even with this trust, it is still important to monitor them, however, as our young people are all vulnerable to peer pressure and are prime targets for brands, as they are the ultimate consumers. Not only do our children have a monopoly on parent pester power, they are also future consumers, and so cultivating their brand loyalty now means a constant money source for these companies in future. Knowledge and awareness is empowering when it comes to technology.

> You have to feed your mind daily with the good, clean, pure, powerful and positive. Feeding your mind is just as important as feeding your body!

Zig Ziglar

I have to admit that it makes my heart sink when I ask a group of 11-12 year-olds if they watch soaps. They all throw their hands up in the air declaring how great this one and that one is, who is cheating on who, who has been murdered, and so forth. I leave it to you to think about the effects of those storylines, particularly when many children think this is what being an adult is really like.

I place no judgements here on what television programmes, social media, games, etc, people choose to spend their time on. I am simply making it known that some things expand the brain and promote happiness, and others can really skew people's idea of reality and promote a dark cloud of negativity.

I have no scientific evidence that watching specific TV programmes had any influence on my own dark days as a teen, but I can tell you that eliminating soaps and sensationalist news from my life has definitely promoted my happiness levels. My children have never been introduced to soaps and I feel glad of that. Studies show that it is difficult for a child to comprehend the difference between real life and fiction before the age of 12, whether it be advertisements, films or programmes. It is a societal norm for children to watch soaps and so please do not feel bad if this is a habit in your household. It is difficult to change habits and so it would be a worthwhile experiment to set the challenge of avoiding a soap for a week and then continuing to avoid it, while replacing it with a new habit. Take note of your child's positivity levels and maybe yours too.

## Encourage critical thinking

Our youth are the perfect target audience for a large percentage of commercial advertising as their brains are under major development. This affects the decision-making and critical thinking parts of the brain, which results in impulsive, rash thinking that can leave them vulnerable. Recent research indicates that children cannot think in an abstract way, critically engage, or question effectively until they reach adolescence (*http://www.adassoc.org.uk/wp-content/uploads/2014/09/Children-and-commercial-communications-A-literature-review.pdf page 22).

At this point habits are set, their taste buds may be defective and they may already be a lifetime consumer of the product!

Listening to a conversation recently, I heard that a man was dismayed at the exorbitant price of a plain pair of trainers, simply because it was emblazoned with the particular brand logo of a company that sells a sugary solution, an example of brilliant marketing!

We already know that many food and drink companies target young people as their future consumers and, of course, pester power is a strong factor in parents' buying decisions. Who doesn't want an easy life occasionally? However, these businesses spend millions of pounds to be good at this, and we are so busy we generally do not have time to pay much attention to these sales tactics. It is something, however, that we need to discuss with our children if we want them to become savvy consumers who are able to make informed decisions. I could give you so many examples from my experiences as a parent, either in school, during my visits to parliament or from my nutrition networking. However, this true story I am about to share with you confirms the priorities of advertising, as discussed in this chapter.

Billboards are placed along the road outside the academy where I teach and recently, much to my dismay, fast food adverts were placed there. Although I understand we cannot control everything and it is important to educate our children to think critically, I feel strongly that companies should not be overtly marketing at a place so close to a school, and so I spoke to a lady at the billboard company in question. She was friendly and extremely approachable, going out of her way to request a prohibition notice. She seemed to be fulfilling her promise of a high sugar/fast food marketing ban but a few short weeks later, there it was – a huge poster for one of the largest junk food companies. I rang my new billboard friend who said she was as confused as I was and promised to investigate and get right back to me. I know I shouldn't have been surprised by her response, but it still shocked me when she confessed that because this was one of their highest-paying clients, who had asked for specific locations, they could not stand by the promised prohibition. Here's what she said:

*"While (business name) do our utmost to respect the wishes of businesses in the locale, such as the academy, please be advised some campaigns are site-specific and cannot be removed as this will lead to a loss of revenue and potential damage to relationships with our clients. I am hoping the prohibitions will stand and there should be no more adverts for fast food or other 'unhealthy' brands posted alongside the school."*

As I write, this is still an ongoing issue. Food preferences are determined mainly by taste. Eating habits and taste preference develop early in life and remain pretty unchanged in adolescence. As taste preferences are acquired through learning, including repeated exposure and messaging about foods, exposure to TV and so on, absorbing these advertisements early in life can have a marked lifelong influence on eating practices. This really is food for thought when we often hear parents or schools being blamed in the battle of healthy food vs. junk.

We are being sold to all of the time, so finding a way to encourage and develop critical thinking in our children is essential if we want to empower them to make their own informed decisions. So, how can we do this?

Discuss advertisements with your child and explain what the companies do to persuade customers to buy. Simply being honest and spending time communicating with your child about your decisions and, of course, modelling your food choices will be much more important than any marketing tactic in the long run. I often explain to students that the food companies are not the bad guys, they are simply making money, as is any other business. However, they do not have our children's health or best interests at heart, as we do.

When you come across marketing on the Internet, unpick it together with your teen and ask them what they think about how companies are persuading people to buy. If nothing else, it may turn them into a marketing genius!

**LINKS**

http://www.child-encyclopedia.com/child-nutrition/
according-experts/television-tv-and-tv-advertisement-
influences-childrens-eating

# Cultivating compassion and gratitude

Anything you do repeatedly becomes a habit. If you understand this, as well as how to establish a new habit, you will have cracked the code to achieving your goals, whether they be related to health, business or any other area of life. Unfortunately for us, parents have accumulated the baggage of programmed habits for many years and although being persistent can change them gradually, establishing habits that serve our children better at an earlier stage has to be a better option; or at least that is my theory.

Albert Schweitzer

> We are what we repeatedly do.
> Excellence, then, is not an act, but a habit.

Every choice we make matters. Choosing to do something healthy over and over again will set you up for good energy levels and overall health. On the flip side, a consequence will ensue if we choose to do something unhealthy on a consistent basis. This could be choosing to go to bed late and sleeping less, which will affect our concentration and energy levels, or choosing to eat an extra biscuit each day, which over time results in weight gain or the opposite effect when you choose to cut out that biscuit altogether. It is often the small things that count. The habit of kindness is no different, it can be developed and nurtured.

As we have already discussed, the teenage years are a tricky time for the human brain. Therefore, anything we can do to support the development of positive traits will benefit you. This can take a little bit of work at first, as you listen out for teen's kind acts towards others. If you are already finding communication with your child a challenge, this can be difficult, but not impossible.

Here is what to do. Tell your adolescent, or someone else in your family or group of friends, that you are proud of them when they help you, and that being kind to others is the most important thing they can do. I feel that by placing more value on acts of kindness than anything else, including their academic success, will strengthen your child's self-esteem and ethical values, as well as promote compassion and gratitude, as what one gives, one will sooner or later receive.

Have you noticed how good it feels when you give a gift, do something for someone or brighten their day? The hormone oxytocin is the reason for this and Theodore Malloch explains in his book Being Generous that giving to others provides us with a sense of connection, which is essential for overall well-being.

I love to talk about 'shining your light' with my children and students. There are many ways we are able to give to others every day - it could be simply by smiling, giving someone a hug who needs it, or helping a friend to get through a challenge by listening and simply being there. Each one of us is unique and we should never underestimate our power to help others feel better. So, go out and shine your light, it feels so good and it will rub off on your teen. I often strike up a conversation with staff at shops and restaurants and have been known to search out the store manager to let them know about a particularly helpful member of staff. Being grateful creates such positivity for both parties and when your children are around, they will replicate this. After seeing how much you get from showing your kindness and gratitude, they will flourish and treat others with respect. It really blows my mind to think of a world where kindness and serving others becomes the focus of every day, as we remember our connection to each other. Every person you meet today wants the exact same things as you do, including love, respect and care.

Here are a few strategies that can help you to cultivate compassion and gratitude in your adolescent, because a lovely side effect of kindness is happiness.

A good way to raise awareness of the kind acts that your child does during their day, and also to encourage further compassion, is to ask this question at the dinner table, or in the conversation you have at the end of the day: "What did you do to help someone today or brighten someone else's day?"

This is a great exercise because we all underestimate our ability to help others to feel good, and yet a smile, a hug, or a few words of encouragement can change everything. This question helps your child to remember they are love and goodness, and they have a lot to give to the world.

Each morning, encourage your child to think of three things they are grateful for before they get up. We call this our thank yous and it is much easier to cultivate before the age of 10. Don't worry too much if it is not taken up immediately. Your teen may prefer to write their gratitude or feelings in a journal at their preferred time of the day. This really works to help them shift to a positive mindset.

I am sure there are many other ways you can encourage kindness in your family. Usually, the ones your children think of are the best. One day, my youngest daughter and I were throwing stones in the river. It was such a beautiful evening and we were saying our thank yous when Ava noticed the water rippling outwards each time she threw a stone. We talked about how each time we did something kind or unkind it had a ripple effect. This has become a fun positive ritual we now have. We throw a stone and shout a loving comment about a friend, family member or situation and watch with laughter as it ripples out, spreading the kindness.

---

Reference: *Being Generous*, a book by Theodore Roosevelt Malloch

## Morning routine

Your child's first greeting can really shape the rest of the day, so how can you make sure it is positive? Establish a routine for waking up your child, which you have agreed together. For example, set a time that you will enter the room and gently kiss your teen on the top of their head and tell them it's 5 minutes to wake up. Encourage them to use this 5 minutes thinking about what they are grateful for. Of course, every adolescent is different and this may not be something your child is open to, particularly in the later teenage years.

## Sleep routine

Take the time to discuss how a sleep routine is important for your teen's brain development as it will enable them to do well in school and prevent them from feeling tired, moody or becoming ill. There is also value in using the old 'beauty sleep' adage, as adolescents care deeply about their appearance. Sleep is the time when we recover and repair, so going to bed at a similar time each night, having been away from any technology for at least an hour before bed, will surely evolve into good sleeping habits.

## Daytime activity

Being active each day will support your teen's mental health and reduce the risk of depression or anxiety. Encourage your child to rise earlier, so that they are not rushing out of the door feeling stressed about being late for school or college. A small routine of stretching, a morning walk, run or cycle, is a perfect way to start the day and get the positive endorphins going. If you have a morning routine, you will find little resistance from your teen. They will see the positive impact on you.

I like to rise early, as this is the quietest time of the day. It's my time to listen, read, stretch, run and write, and my girls know my routine. Last year when my daughter turned 13, she started to rise earlier to do a short YouTube yoga routine. I did not tell her to do this, she just saw that my morning time energised me and now loves to run through the village, or go for walks appreciating that time to herself.

# Chapter 7

# Nourish your teen

> Let food be thy medicine...
>  Hippocrates

Incorporating a healthy lifestyle can be a challenge if you, as a parent, haven't had the scene set in your own upbringing. However, believe me, following simple steps for feeding your whole family will pay dividends for their health. Good nutrition reduces illness, supports positive learning behaviours, reduces irritability, supports healthy skin and promotes positive mental well-being.

I teach teens to cook from scratch and use a variety of flavours and ingredients. My own diet as a teen consisted of large amounts of junk food, which I am now sure contributed to my poor mental health. You can make a change anytime. Take it slow and know that you deserve to feel good and nourish yourself with natural foods. Perfection is not the goal, a little bit of junk is not so harmful to your teen if their daily diet is overflowing with nutritious foods.

It is quite usual to have up to a quarter of my class state their initial dislike of a specific ingredient, such as tomatoes or onions, in food lessons. I want my students to understand that taste is not static, it is changeable and acquired. So I explain they can gain the health benefits of an ingredient by tasting it a number of times or disguising it in special ways, which we discuss. I grew up convinced that I did not like tomatoes, but as soon as I studied the lycopene content, a powerful antioxidant with the ability to inhibit cancer cell growth, I started to add them to everything. Funnily enough, I now absolutely love them.

There is so much evidence to show that taste preferences are acquired or learned and they can be adjusted. So if you are coming up against resistance, be patient and keep offering your child foods and encourage them to prepare and/or cook dinner with you. Cooking together is a perfect time to engage in conversation and listen to your teen, as it helps to pull down their defences. If your teen is not interested in getting involved in the kitchen, make it one of their chores, but keep it simple at first, so as not to overwhelm them. I find that pupils who are trusted in their kitchen at home have a higher degree of confidence and belief in themselves when cooking in school. My more nervous students usually say things like, "My mum says I am a disaster in the kitchen," or "I am not trusted to put things in the oven."

Teach your adolescent safety first, e.g. always use an oven glove, check there is no one close by, fully open the oven door, and then trust them to get on with it. Yes, your kitchen will be messy to start with and it will take practice for them to multitask and keep it clean as they go along. But I assure you, by trusting them and gradually allowing them to help, this will promote their self-esteem and make your life so much easier. My teen is able to produce the most delicious meals and, being a working mum, my appreciation for this holds no limits. You will find Abigail's signature recipes in my healthy recipe (download available at http://passionatenutrition. co.uk/).

> Cooking from scratch is the single most important thing we could do as a family to improve our health and general well-being.

Michael Pollan

A further point to note here regarding children's tastes is that they are being sold to from the moment they wake up each day (as previously discussed in Chapter 5), which has affected our society's whole way of eating. Vegetables have become an object of disdain and parents have had to find creative ways of hiding them in sauces and even cakes! The more we eat processed foods produced by companies that have perfected the 'bliss point', the less our taste buds are willing to consume natural foods. This 'bliss point was uncovered and documented by the journalist Michael Moss in his book, Salt, Sugar, Fat: How the Food Giants Hooked Us. Health messages can be confusing and the best example of this is the 'low fat' phenomenon, as we now understand that it is not beneficial to take fat completely out of our diet. However, the campaigns to 'eat more vegetables' have always been clear - eating more vegetables will result in an increased quality of health, better skin and less risk of numerous illnesses and diseases.

> Eat food, not too much, mostly plants.

Michael Pollan

## Essential breakfast

Breakfast for young people is essential, in my opinion, as it ensures your child starts the day with an energy supply to the body and brain. This influx of nutrients supports concentration and learning.

It is always best to avoid sugary products, otherwise your child will be sent on a blood sugar spike rollercoaster. This can cause irritability, which has an impact on not only their learning, but also their relationships. This is before we even get into tooth decay and muffin tops (fat accumulation around the waist). How our bodies metabolise sugar is a cause for great concern. This includes refined flours and carbohydrates lacking in fibre (as fibre slows the insulin spikes), such as white bread, bagels or muffins, which initiate a boost of energy only to quickly cause a crash in blood sugars, causing the aforementioned symptoms of irritability and moodiness.

**A breakfast strategy:**
The aim of breakfast is to provide the fuel that your adolescent needs to get through the morning. This will establish a healthy habit for life, give them the energy to do all that they want to do and enable them to concentrate well. To achieve this, the basics of breakfast must include healthy fats, protein and slow release complex carbohydrates. Adding fruits and/or vegetables will add extra nutrients that support optimum health for immunity and overall body and skin health. The recipes and plan at the end of the book will provide you with a good basis for a healthy energy boost at the start of the day.

## Mealtimes

We have already discussed the advantages of cooking together, as it involves your teen in the cooking process. However, it is also important because it provides a safe platform for listening and conversation, promoting self-esteem and trust, and also teaching your teen about different ingredients and meal planning.

Traditionally, we were taught to think about the meat first, then potatoes/pasta/rice, and then lastly to sneak a few veggies in there for luck. However, high rates of cancer and cardiovascular disease in areas where the Western diet prevails indicate that we are getting it wrong. Take a leaf out of the Blue Zones principles devised by Dan Buettner, which recommend reducing animal produce, eating more vegetables and snacking on fruit, nuts and seeds. This is much easier than following a diet that requires hours of weighing, working out our blood type, or whether it is a protein or a green day. Gosh, it is enough to put you off trying to cook for a family!

## My simple evening meal planning strategy

My clients and friends often express their frustration at not knowing where to start and think that when they are working and busy, adopting new things takes too much time. So here is my simple evening meal planning strategy for all busy parents.

**Step 1:** Start by thinking about which vegetables you will use. Have three or four varieties at each meal; for example, a chilli could include carrots, onions, courgettes and mushrooms, not to mention garlic, chilli and tomatoes.

**Step 2:** Add protein, such as lentils, chickpeas, beans, or a small amount of organic meat or fish.

**Step 3:** Add starchy carbohydrates – a fist-sized portion of wholemeal, spelt or rice pasta, couscous, brown rice, baked potato or sweet potato wedges/mash.

**Step 4:** Add healthy fats, either for cooking or to use as a dressing. For example, olive, coconut or avocado oil (avocado is very stable at high heat and so this may be the best option for cooking), avocado and seeds contain healthy fats, which can be added to meals.

## Portion sizes

Portion sizes are often blamed for contributing to the obesity epidemic and, therefore, this is a handy, easy-to-use guide to what's appropriate.

Make a habit of serving a fist-sized portion of starchy carbohydrates (your child's own fist size for their portion), plus a thumb-sized portion of fats and a palm-sized portion of protein.

The good news is that veggies can be piled on for your teens, just go for a good variety of colours.

## Aim for progress, not perfection

I know it is not always easy to eat together and have healthy meals set for every evening, but it can be simple once you know how. Having all the ingredients ready to use is just one way to be prepared. For example, you could chop ginger into thumb-sized pieces or dice garlic and onions and then store them in the freezer. You could make a big batch of soup and freeze it into smaller portions for busy evenings, or pre-roast the veggies so they are ready to warm up and add to a tomato-based sauce. Some evenings, it may be omelette and salad with fruit at supper. This is very quick and easy, but extremely nutritious.

The best approach is not to do everything all at once. Remember, progress and not perfection is the key. Introduce one new meal that meets the principles that we've already discussed, every week for a month, and then another. Before you know it, you will have a plant-based approach to evening meals. (You will find more ideas in my free recipe book, which you can download at: http://passionatenutrition.co.uk/.)

## The importance of eating together

Eating regular meals together with at least one parent, at least five times a week, is beneficial to young people, as this seems to reduce the risk of teenage pregnancy, depression, eating disorders and high risk-taking behaviours, e.g. drug and alcohol abuse. Therefore, it seems to have an impact on increasing your child's self-esteem and helps to build resilience, as well as boosting their vocabulary and academic success. My feeling is that it comes back to at least one of our three Cs: communication.

Dr Anne K Fishel, who is a cofounder of The Family Dinner Project and author of *Home for Dinner*, explains that sharing a family meal is good for the spirit, the brain and the health of all the family. When you take all of these things into account, it is clear what a difference eating with your family can make.

As parents of teens, we know how it feels to be grunted at, and you sometimes need to be canny to get around this, especially as your teen may misread your facial signals and fly off the handle at your confusion… Good nutrition can really help to reduce the irritability effect, as can asking the right question at the dinner table. Ever since my children were small, I have asked a similar question, which is: "Anything interesting happen today?"

For some unknown reason, it works. When you ask, "What did you do today?" more often than not, the response will be, "I don't know", if you're lucky. However, the 'anything interesting?' approach seems to get them thinking and their news about the day starts to flood out, as if they are searching for the interesting thing that may have happened.

Conversation starters are always good at dinner as they seem to take the pressure off asking too many questions for teens (you know how they hate too many questions). For example:

*"If you could go absolutely anywhere around the world right now, where would you go and why?"*
*"What are you most excited about today?"*
*"What is the kindest thing you did today?"*
*"If you could ask a question to anyone in the world, who would you ask and what would it be?"'*

This is really fun and you get some interesting responses. They usually want to know what your response would be, and so it becomes a shared discussion that inadvertently teaches your children the art of conversation.

## LINKS

http://thefamilydinnerproject.org/resources/faq/

## How do our bodies metabolise sugar and why is it a problem?

I always had a sweet tooth and thought that it was just a part of my life until a few years ago, but it doesn't have to be, and although we are naturally hard-wired to seek out sweet things, having them available for 24 hours a day is certainly a different matter. It really concerns me when I see young people who think nothing of replacing their meals with sweets, sugar for breakfast, a packet of biscuits for tea and sweets in between. Oh, and let's add in a few energy drinks. Besides it being extremely detrimental to our teeth, too much sugar can have dire consequences for our physical, mental health and well-being.

All of the carbohydrates you ingest from fruits, vegetables, starches, grains and the other sugars are broken down into simple sugars taken into the blood. This influx elevates the blood sugar. The hormone insulin is then released to allow the sugar, which is broken down into glucose and fructose, into your cells and to be used for energy. When the insulin requirement is increased due to a high intake of sugary products, a signal is created to store these extra calories for leaner times (sugar is converted into fat, aka the muffin top). When you take in a lot of free/simple sugars at once, the insulin levels rise rapidly, leading to a sudden crash in blood sugars. The sudden dip indicates you are low on fuel and this causes you to feel hungry in an effort to increase your blood sugars again. Furthermore, if your blood sugar suddenly drops, it can lead to many physical and mental symptoms, such as dizziness, headaches, nausea, blurred vision, sweating, palpitations, cravings and irritability. This is common when you skip meals or miss breakfast if you are someone who often consumes simple sugars.

It is easy to see how this becomes a cycle of overeating and craving sugary foods which results in yo-yoing insulin levels. When you eat wholefood sources of carbohydrates (vegetables and fruits), together with healthy fats and protein, the glucose from the food enters our blood gradually, and the pancreas secretes an adequate quantity of insulin.

Note that fat accumulating around the middle causes a sluggish clearing of blood sugar. This leads to insulin resistance and can, in turn, potentially lead to type 2 diabetes because the pancreas becomes exhausted and is unable to produce sufficient quantities of insulin.

I share this information with you because an awareness about of how sugar impacts our bodies can support you in reducing the amount of free sugars that you and your family consume. Hidden sugars can also be a problem, so a good tip is to look for food products that have 5g or less of sugar per 100g.

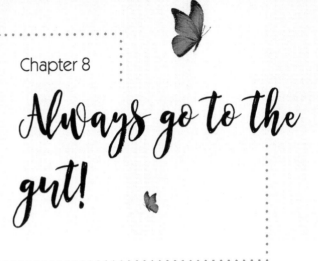

Chapter 8

# Always go to the gut!

If your child has a cold or a minor illness, this chapter may support you. Contrary to our learned Western thinking, which leads us to buy over-the-counter remedies, let your thoughts initially go to your child's gut health. For centuries Chinese, Indian and herbal traditions have made digestive health a priority. There is always a place for Western medicine and I am not advocating replacing Western medicine altogether. However, it is useful long-term to try natural methods and food as medicine first.

All disease begins in the gut.  Hippocrates

Our human cells live in a symbiotic relationship with 100 trillion microorganisms, which we know as our microbiome, or what I like to call our 'gut garden'. We have more bacteria living on our skin and in our gut than we have human cells. It stands to reason, then, that keeping our bacteria happy and healthy will improve our overall health.

Scientists have already found that increased hygiene and cleanliness has led to an escalation in infectious diseases, with a significant increase in allergies and autoimmune diseases. Interestingly, studies have also shown that children who come in contact with farm animals develop fewer allergies during their lifetime. Further studies that involved administering antibiotics to baby mice showed that a loss of beneficial bacteria increases the incidences of allergies. So, if your teen has an allergy, intolerance or coeliac, I encourage you to focus on improving their gut health, whilst also removing the allergen from their diet.

## Gut-brain connection

Certain strains of probiotics can increase the availability of tryptophan, the key precursor to making serotonin. There is already - and I am sure there will be further - evidence to prove the gut-brain connection. Serotonin, the hormone that every prescription drug for depression taps into, is available from all plants. The disruption to this essential hormone comes from stress, chemicals, technology and food additives. This is why eating wholefoods and a high fibre diet, including lots of fruit and vegetables, may dramatically improve a person's health if they are ill, suffer from autoimmunity issues or have mental health conditions.

Furthermore, the bacteria in our body may also influence our genes, so promoting good bacteria can only be a positive move.

So what can you do?

- Reduce processed foods, junk foods and sugar
- Eat more fibre from fruit and vegetables
- Consume fist-sized portions of wholegrain starchy carbohydrates, e.g. spelt pasta, brown or black rice
- Eat fermented foods, such as miso paste, tamari (in place of soy sauce), sauerkraut and kimchi
- Consume fermented drinks as much as possible. You can buy kefir water and kombucha from some health shops or online
- Most importantly, consume lots of greens and fibrous vegetables, including onions, garlic, leeks, etc.
- Take a high quality probiotic, either in a powder form or capsule

## LINKS

http://academicminute.org/2016/03/jack-gilbert-university-of-chicago-diversifying-your-microbiome/

https://www.psychologytoday.com/blog/evolutionary-psychiatry/201404/the-gut-brain-connection-mental-illness-and-disease

https://www.ncbi.nlm.nih.gov/pmc/articles/PMC3637398/

# Chapter 9

# Nutrients for brain health

I am sure that by the time you reach this chapter you will be aware that eating natural foods and reducing processed food has an impact on our whole body. However, the development of our children's brains is important to us and we want to be able to nourish this particular part of the body.

While the previous chapter was relevant to a healthy thriving brain, this chapter focuses on those particular nutrients that can support a child with a specific need. I shared earlier that my eldest daughter has dyslexic tendencies. These have caused her some distress, although I am proud to note that her resilience and the way she embraces challenges is way beyond what I was capable of as a teen. It seems that the hardship has only strengthened her will. No matter what the challenges are, and there are plenty for every teen, it is beneficial for them to face them head on, knowing that they are something to learn from. This positive attitude will help them to thrive. There is only getting something right or learning, there is no losing or getting it wrong. If you can embrace that with your teen, they can face failures even when they feel frightened.

A varied, natural diet is required for the brain's optimal health and there have been numerous studies that focused on specific nutrients. Nevertheless, it is difficult to find conclusive evidence in many of them that a specific nutrient is effective. Herein, I will focus on the nutrients that have been suggested to improve cognitive function, both in populations that are poorer or have specific learning issues. Supplementation is not out of the question when it comes to boosting and supporting health, but a 'supplement' is just that. It should never be thought of as a replacement for a wholefood.

Zinc, iron, B12 and omega 3 have all been found to support brain health and learning[1]. The list of foods below will allow you to ensure that your teen is getting a range of these nutrients. Supplementing and increasing levels of omega 3 fatty acids in children has also been found to be beneficial, not only for those with SpLD, but also those with poor attention and a low reading ability[2]. Therefore, I feel it is beneficial to make sure you include oily fish or a vegan source of omega 3 from algae, walnuts or flaxseed/linseeds in your teen's diet. In my opinion, the addition of an omega 3 supplement has supported my daughter's learning experience.

> Tip: If you are going to use a fish oil supplement, please ensure that you purchase it from a sustainably aware company. This ensures they have added vitamin E or another antioxidant that prevents the fish oil from going rancid, which would make it ineffective and actually detrimental to health.

It is also important to note here that all nutrients have adversaries, which can deplete or take away our ability to absorb essential nutrients for our health. It is good for our teens to understand that tea, coffee or other sources of caffeine, alcohol and smoking can greatly deplete these nutrients from our bodies, causing poor health, both in the short-term and the long-term.

## Zinc food sources include:

sesame seeds
quinoa
cashew nuts
lentils
pumpkin seeds
beans
shitake and cremini
mushrooms

spinach
asparagus
oats
beef
turkey
peas
broccoli
tomatoes

## Iron food sources include:

kale
watercress
spinach
green peppers
brown rice
kidney beans
peanuts
pistachios
pumpkin seeds
sunflower seeds

sesame seeds
meat
fish
tofu
eggs
dried apricots
dates
raisins
spirulina

## B12 food sources include:

eggs
meat

fish
nutritional yeast

A vegetarian or vegan will find it difficult to gain the levels of B12 they require, particularly if they are not regularly consuming nutritional yeast. Therefore, a supplement is essential. If you do not eat meat and are feeling tired, have sugar cravings and/or experiencing a low mood, it may be beneficial for you to supplement with B12.

## Omega 3 food sources include:

flaxseeds
chia seeds
hemp seeds
algae oil
walnuts
mackerel

salmon
herring
tuna
anchovies
cod liver oil
egg yolks

---

[1] Nutrients for Cognitive Development in School-aged Children, Janet Bryan, Ph.D., Saskia Osendarp, Ph.D., Donna Hughes, MPsych, Eva Calvaresi, MPsych, Katrine Baghurst, Ph.D., and Jan-Willem van Klinken, Ph.D., August 2004: 295-306

http://www.ncbi.nlm.nih.gov/pubmed/23826114

[2] Low blood long chain omega-3 fatty acids in UK children are associated with poor cognitive performance and behavior: a cross-sectional analysis from the DOLAB study. Montgomery P1, Burton JR, Sewell RP, Spreckelsen TF, Richardson AJ.

# Chapter 10

# Nourishment for the menstrual cycle

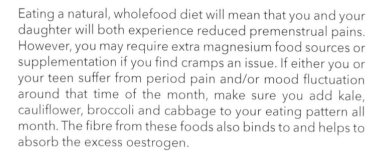

Eating a natural, wholefood diet will mean that you and your daughter will both experience reduced premenstrual pains. However, you may require extra magnesium food sources or supplementation if you find cramps an issue. If either you or your teen suffer from period pain and/or mood fluctuation around that time of the month, make sure you add kale, cauliflower, broccoli and cabbage to your eating pattern all month. The fibre from these foods also binds to and helps to absorb the excess oestrogen.

Magnesium strengthens the bones and teeth whilst promoting healthy muscles, helping them to relax. This means it is important for premenstrual symptoms (PMS), the heart and nervous system, as well as energy production. However, too much animal produce, particularly dairy, wheat and rhubarb, can disrupt the absorption of magnesium and cause you to become deficient in this essential mineral. Many people crave chocolate. This is very interesting as raw cacao (chocolate) is high in magnesium, which also helps with the absorption of calcium.

During the menstrual cycle, the oestrogen fluctuation can affect our calcium absorption. Therefore, consume plenty of green leafy vegetables, broccoli, beans, dried apricots, nuts and seeds, which will increase your calcium intake, along with a small amount of organic red meat (if you eat animal products). Studies show that eating more calcium can reduce the low moods and improve your concentration during the menstrual cycle. (http://www.ncbi.nlm.nih.gov/pubmed/8498421)

Ideally, your teen would consume 2 to 3 portions of fish per week. However, this may not be possible; therefore, take omega 3 in a supplement form (algae for a vegan source/fish oil) every day to alleviate the pain, as omega 3 has been found to reduce inflammation and help balance hormones.

## The importance of iron

Iron deficiency and anaemia is a well-known problem around the world and research shows that our iron requirements nearly double during *adolescence for both males and females. We know now that improved iron status has an impact on learning and is thought to benefit cognitive development. This essential mineral has so many jobs within the human body, it is no wonder that being low in iron adversely affects our overall health. It is a vital component in red blood cells and the enzymes are used in energy, protein and hormone production.

The UK Dietary Reference Values (DRVs) provide guidance on the quantity of iron we need to consume to meet our body's needs. It is suggested that taking more than 17mg is too much (NHS, 2017), unless prescribed by a doctor. The DRV for a male is 8.7mg per day and 14.8mg for a female. Note that high doses of iron from supplements can be fatal, so it is important to keep them out of reach from children and seek medical advice.

## Dietary iron, blockers and supporters

Dietary iron is found in meat, as haem-iron, and cereals, vegetables, nuts, pulses, eggs, fish and meat, as non-haem iron. There is much to learn about how much iron we require and how it is absorbed. We know, for example, that phytic acid, which is found in whole-grain, nuts, seeds, soya and pulses, disturbs the absorption of iron in our bodies, as do polyphenols found in *black tea, coffee, cocoa and red wine. Calcium sourced in such products as milk and cheese is also found to inhibit the absorption of this important mineral is. However, research has shown that vitamin C (ascorbic acid) supports the absorption of iron. Therefore, it would be highly beneficial to include a good source of vitamin C from fruit and vegetables with all your meals.

## Are vegetarians more likely to be low in iron?

If you or your child do not consume meat, then this alone should not have a significant impact on your iron levels, contrary to popular belief. Vegetarian diets tend to have higher intakes of non-haem iron and also higher intakes of foods that include phytates (the inhibitors). However, the research indicates that both vegetarians and non-vegetarians have a similar iron status (SACN, 2010). Therefore, not eating meat is not a problem, as long as a varied diet is eaten. There needs to be a high intake of vitamin C and reduced intake of inhibitors that will support a good iron status.

LINKS

**SACN, 2010, Iron and health:**
https://www.gov.uk/government/uploads/system/uploads/attachment_data/file/339309/SACN_Iron_and_Health_Report.pdf
(accessed 26 February 2017)

**Beard, J.L., Iron Requirements in Adolescent females, Journal of Nutrition, February 1, 2000 vol. 130 no. 2 440S-442S** http://jn.nutrition.org/content/130/2/440S.full.pdf+html (accessed 26 February 2017)

**NHS, 2017, Iron** http://www.nhs.uk/Conditions/vitamins-minerals/Pages/Iron.aspx (accessed 26 February 2017)

---

* John Beard's review of iron requirements in adolescent females in 2000 found that "diminished iron stores are likely in a significant proportion of adolescent females in developed and developing countries". In addition, there seems to be a lack of opportunity to improve iron levels in many cases for the requirements of a healthy pregnancy (Beard, 2000).

* The impact of phytates on iron absorption can be improved by vitamin C (ascorbic acid) and meat consumption (Hallberg et al, 1989; Siegenberg et al, 1991). Hallberg et al (1989) estimated that approximately 80 mg of ascorbic acid would be needed to counteract the inhibitory effect of 25 mg of phytate P, and that very large amounts (several hundred mg) would be required to overcome the inhibitory effects of high phytate diets (SACN, 2010).

* Coffee has approximately half the inhibitory effect of tea, although black tea is a more powerful inhibitor than herbal tea, cocoa or wine. 50 mg of ascorbic acid was required to overcome the effects of >100 mg tannic acid (SACN, 2010).

# Chapter 11

# Embracing your body shape

You may feel your teen may has the most perfect body shape, but if you are unhappy about your own shape, they will feel it. I have heard parents remark how disgusting they feel their body is when they show it in front of their child. This will damage your child's view of itself, even though you would never want this to happen. You are unique and important and your birth was a miracle, just like your teen's was.

Spend time affirming the gift of your body. If you are unhappy with it and talk about yourself negatively, your teen will almost certainly pick this up. The fact you are reading this book means you want your child to be self-assured and happy, and I know what I'm asking is not easy to do, but if you embrace your body, warts and all, this will result in your teen accepting theirs.

I didn't always feel comfortable in my own skin and when I had the girls, I knew that I didn't want them to feel the same painful self-loathing that I did. Nutrition and personal growth took on a whole new meaning as a result of my gorgeous girls coming into my life, and so it became my mission and passion. I was determined they would find their way to self-acceptance and now, through my search, I can share with you the knowledge that the only way is to learn self-love*.

At first, faking it is the best way. I have danced with my girls, declaring my gratitude for curves while we wiggle our bottoms with glee. The wonderful thing about this is that you wake up one day after affirming it for so long and actually believe it!

* See the self-love formula page.

# Chapter 12

# Navigating friendships, hurt and emotional times

Encourage a good variety of friendships and discourage the 'one best friend' is all I need phenomenon (which is so common, I assure you) as early as you can. It is painful when we see our children hurt after falling out with their friends and in the majority of cases (unless there is a bullying issue) it is much better to stay out of it and allow them to work things out. After all, in Marianne Williams' words, it is part of their 'curriculum'. They are learning and they will make mistakes, as they are imperfect too. Trust is important because we can worry about the company that our teens choose to keep; however, if we work at all of the three Cs, we will provide our teens with a good moral grounding to make their own decisions. A strong sense of self-esteem will result in them staying away from risk-taking behaviours and those who want to participate in them.

There will undoubtedly be emotional times, as falling out with friends, arguments, sadness over a friend moving away, the death of a pet or grief over the loss of a family member are real-life situations. These are all huge, confusing challenges for your child and they will look to you and need your support, except for the times when they may react by emotionally pushing you away. This is just another opportunity for open communication and to show them how to be a good listener and empathise. As I keep noting, you are being observed, even if it's only subconsciously. Just like you, your teen wants to be listened to, and a good way to reassure them you are listening is to gently state the obvious. For example, by saying, "You seem upset," or "This has made you feel sad, hasn't it?" Then you can share a past situation when you felt like they do right now. Doing this demonstrates empathy and helps them to feel like they are not being judged or what they are going through is not unusual.

Allow or plan in some alone time for your child to read, play, draw etc. from an early age, while cultivating their self-esteem. Letting them see that your alone time is important as well will reduce the 'I need attention 24-7 syndrome' and promote self-assurance. Your teen's self-esteem must be preserved. I am certainly not a scaremonger, but this is the time when mental health issues can develop. In fact, half of all lifetime cases are reported to have begun by the age of 14.

You can certainly reduce the risk of mental health issues for your teen because, after all, they want what we all want – to be listened to and loved (not to mention the natural eating and our bacteria we have already covered). They can make doing these things a little more difficult, as they are not always able to convey their wants, and are often in a state of emotional confusion due to their hormonal imbalances or brain redevelopment. I am no stranger to teen tantrums and the pulling of faces. For a little while, I thought my eldest daughter had lost all of her personality and the ability to smile. I wasn't always patient through these times and luckily the personality transplant was very short-lived. However, when I did react without compassion, I apologised. This always opens up the communication lines with your child and enables them to tell you what is going on. Sometimes, they don't even know themselves; they just feel angry or upset. Being there for them is really all you need to do.

This is all part of embracing your imperfection, so show your teen it is OK to make mistakes and how to communicate. No one ever said parenting was easy, but always remember that sticking with them in the short-term will make both your life and theirs better in the long run. To help you keep on track, revisit the third C, 'communication', and make sure that you know what is going on in your teen's life. What are they happy and excited about and what is stressing them? Let them know you are on their side and you love them unconditionally.

**LINKS**

//www.nimh.nih.gov/news/science-news/2005/mental-illness-exacts-heavy-toll-beginning-in-youth.shtml

## The importance of saying 'no' and sticking to it

When my girls were little, I used to tell them that it was hard to say no to them, but it was part of being a good mummy. I explained that saying 'no' firmly and sticking to the decision would stop them from being like Veruca Salt in the story of Charlie and the Chocolate Factory. This slightly fairy-tale explanation always appeased them and lightened the impact of my 'no', helping them to understand, albeit comically, why boundaries are important.

I will never tire of listening to Zig Ziglar's view on parenting and have listened to Raising Positive Kids in a Negative World a number of times. Zig talks about times when he has said 'no' to the requests of his children to attend a party or a friend's get together. Although his daughter was at first frustrated and angry with him, she was actually relieved after he explained why he did not want her going to a particular place. His children often used their father's refusal as a good excuse not to take part in high-risk behaviours. This is such a true phenomenon; our teens may sulk and scream with frustration at being told they cannot do X, Y and Z, but as long as you have their best interests at heart and a good reason to say 'no', they will calm down. You can then explain you are putting their safety first and you love them, and they will understand (eventually). They may even thank you one day! Again, be prepared for a little pain now in order to spare you a lot of pain later.

## When to say 'yes'

Know that being there for your teen and holding space in a non-judgemental way for your teen to practise flying, such as making mistakes and learning, is essential in the process of allowing your child to fulfil their own soul purpose. Allowing for these things and saying 'yes' in as many situations as possible is important. This sounds contradictory to the last section, but I assure you, this is about getting out of the comfort zones to promote confidence and the development of self-love by, for example, having adventures and not indulging in high risk-taking behaviours that damage self-esteem.

The phenomenon of saying 'yes' can be just as challenging to some parents as saying 'no' is to others, as parents can keep saying 'no' to avoid making the wrong decision. If this sounds familiar to you, practice saying 'yes'. As you are asked about a situation, think and ask yourself the following questions:

1. Will this activity pose any long-term risk to my child's self-esteem?
2. Does the danger outweigh the development in this situation?
3. Will my teen be challenged and stretched in a developmental way?
4. Is this desire to say 'no' a result of my own fears?

I will give you a recent example when I made a very unpopular decision without the support of those around me.

When my daughter turned 14 last summer, she was offered a marvellous opportunity by a teacher to travel to her holiday home in Spain and stay with a French-speaking family. Although I knew the teacher was a most wonderful lady, as I worked with her at the same school, I had not met her family and didn't know where she lived. I discussed the trip with my daughter, who was excited and absolutely desperate to go, but the rest of our family tried to persuade me against the trip, saying it was a bad idea. I knew it was a fantastic opportunity and my instincts were to allow her to go, and so I booked her on a Skyflyer Solo flight, much to the disapproval of some disgruntled but well-meaning relatives. She enjoyed the most amazing cultural experience. If I had given in to other people's fears, it would have never happened. I had to weigh up the options and book the safest travelling package to ensure the risk was minimal. In this case, the development and experience far outweighed the danger. We must try and set our fears and ego aside in order to allow our children to fly and fulfil their potential.

# Chapter 13

## Developing Self-respect

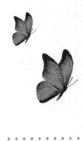

When your teen starts to demonstrate moodiness or a perceived personality change, as I referred to earlier, you must not allow them to pull you down or be disrespectful towards you. I have seen teens and much younger children do this. The parent is looking for an easy life, thinking that 'kids will be kids', and believes that ignoring the behaviour is the best policy. There is also the very good advice that we should not give too much attention to poor behaviour. Although there is truth in that, it is also important to stop a behaviour being carried out if it is disrespectful to all of those involved.

I completely agree that we should never engage in a battle because as soon as this happens we have lost the war. However, your teen must be told authoritatively that you will not put up with cheek or rudeness simply because you are their parent/guardian. They must be told you have their best interests at heart and deserve the same respect you give them. It may be that you need to practise a stern 'don't mess with me' voice if it doesn't come naturally. When you say this, you are not entering into an argument, as being firm in this way is very different to arguing with your child. Standing in your power in certain circumstances is what is needed, and a warm, reasoning conversation can follow later when the time is right. Think back to your own childhood; what would you say worked with you? I always think it is interesting that young people often say a teacher was their favourite because of their firm but fair attitude.

A call for respect from a mother figure who is standing their ground will reduce disrespectful behaviour and also instil self-respect in themselves. Remember, your teen is watching and absorbing your every move, so if you preserve your self-respect, they will follow suit.

# Chapter 14

# Using praise to enthuse and inspire

As a teacher, I know the power of praise; I see it on a daily basis. Finding a specific positive about what and how a student is performing can initiate a strong motivation to do well. I also know that I also respond well to positive feedback. Think about it, it gives you a real boost and a sense of satisfaction. Not only does genuine praise motivate, but it also energises and promotes good self-esteem. Dr David Hamilton, the author, speaker and blogger, talks about his time as a sports coach. Although he was not trained to take on the role, David tapped into what made him tick when he was a youngster, and guess what it was? Yes – praise! He found that 'it' significantly improved performance more than anything else.

This is a good time to discuss giving your teen responsibility around the house and providing them with a chance to learn the lesson of earning cash. It is preferable to start gradually with small jobs, such as dusting, setting the table, etc., before your child reaches the teenage years. However, teens do tend to need/want more things that money can buy, so tying household chores to a weekly allowance is a good way to get them to stick to their chores. Write down the job list, just as you may have done on a sticker chart when they were younger, and make sure they are clear about what they are to do. The completion of chores well done is an ideal opportunity to praise them and will encourage them to want to keep up the great work. Please note, do not praise your child for a half-hearted attempt. Make sure you are firm and refuse to pay unless the job has been completed satisfactorily. Set these expectations early on and your teen will learn. Avoid the 'Oh, I will just do it myself' approach. This is the 'anything for an easy life' syndrome and it will not help you or them in the long run. As an important add-on to this, I have found that self-esteem is greatly boosted when your teen knows how much they have helped you out. For example, my eldest daughter is a fantastic cook and prepares, cooks and serves dinner once or twice a week. As a busy mum, being able to walk in the door and not have to start cooking is the most wonderful feeling, and I make sure I let her know how grateful I am. After all, praise encourages repeat behaviours.

If your child is not academically gifted, achievement praise can seem to be a challenge because of the way that our education system, for the most part, is framed. I earlier shared with you my daughter's gift; however, as my daughter started school it was clear she did not fit in with 'average educational expectations'. I was told how lovely and verbally bright my daughter was at every parents evening, but how she 'struggled' in reading, spelling, etc. I wasn't aware of dyslexia and she had not been assessed at that time, all I knew was that my daughter was happy and interested in all that was going on around her, so I vowed that she would develop self-esteem by trying other things. I became determined to encourage her independence and self-esteem in other ways if our education system was not up to the task.

Well, she took part in nearly every workshop, hobby or activity in our town! She started and stopped things, such as swimming for a while, but has stuck with her love of horses and come back to her love of drama for the most part. But it didn't really matter; it is the diversity that matters and praise for trying new things. This has given her a thirst for adventure and exploration, which is what she loves. She is now so tuned into getting out of her comfort zone and this has boosted her confidence. Furthermore, the fact she has worked harder than those of 'average educational ability' has developed her 'I can do' attitude, which inspires me every day. Here, the moral of the story is 'do not let a challenge be an obstacle, let it be the way.'(Sorry, I just couldn't resist this, as The Obstacle is the Way is the title of one my favourite books, written by Ryan Holiday).

So, look for things to praise; it can be too easy to focus on the untidy bedroom, the sulk or teen tantrum. Make it an exercise where you look for one specific thing every day that you can praise your teen for. This is easy to do if you have a specific chores list and you have set clear expectations for them. Do this every day for a week and see the light of motivation appear in your teen.

## Self-confidence formula

I have learned that self-confidence is the key to success and developing it is just a matter of practice. It requires a general reprogramming of the thoughts and stories you have accumulated over the years. The wonderful thing about supporting our teens in developing this is they have a head start. I didn't identify self-confidence as a key to fulfilling our dreams until my mid-thirties, when I read Napoleon Hill's Think and Grow Rich. It would be wonderful to think of teenagers everywhere growing in confidence and understanding the power that is within them right now. They can make a start and do not have to wait until negativity and fear require them to use these reprogramming tactics.

Here is a self-confidence formula that you can read at least once a day, preferably twice, morning and night. You and your teen can do this and reap the rewards. Firstly, encourage your teen to write down an ambition or dream they would like to come true. This may be writing a book, being a famous vlogger, travelling to a specific country, carrying out an adventurous activity/hobby or something else. The, read out this self-confidence formula for the ultimate results:

1. I have the ability to achieve my purpose in life and commit to persistent and consistent daily actions.

2. I know the thoughts most dominant in my mind on a consistent basis will become reality, and so I commit to concentrating on the type of person I want to become, creating a clear visual image of a confident me.

3. I know that any desires and visions that I keep hold of in my mind will seek to be expressed in outer reality. I also commit to believing in my dreams and ambitions by working on developing self-confidence each day.

4.  I have written down a description of my aim in life and I will never stop trying until I have developed sufficient self-confidence for it to happen.

5.  I have full faith in myself and will be truthful, loving and giving to others with a positive attitude, which will bring me success.

6.  I commit to seeing the good in others and myself.

7.  I commit to repeating this formula aloud once a day and know it will influence my thoughts over time, and I will become a self-reliant and successful person.

Adapted from Napoleon Hill, Think and Grow Rich – the self-confidence formula.

## Self-love formula

As I have learned, consistent self-confidence is the key to success and self-love is the key to happiness. This is why no amount of success can make you happy if you do not also have self-love. Again, if you can support your child in developing self-acceptance early in life, the sky's the limit for their happiness and fulfilment. Use this self-love formula daily and incorporate it as a practice.

This may sound a little crazy but it works, so just give it a go. It will become easier, I assure you. Stand in front of the mirror. You can do this without the mirror as you progress, but use it for at least a few weeks as you become fluent in this mantra. When you know the statement off by heart, you can use it anywhere, such as in the car or on the bus, and you can say it out loud or in your head.

**I am love.**
**I am confident.**
**I am grateful to be surrounded by love.**
**I love me, I'm whole and perfect as I was created to be.**
**Thank you, thank you, thank you.**

As you become confident with the mantra, change it to suit you. Add in some more 'I ams' to affirm your positive view of yourself, such as "I am creative."

Both success and self-love formulas work because they focus on reprogramming our thoughts. The power of our mind as a healing method, manifesting our life as our thoughts, has been proved by physics. We are what we think...

## Gratitude practice

Feeling grateful every day leaves very little room for negativity. This is a little strategy that always works. I have used this to help my own children and students feel good and forget their worries. It is called a practice because it is just that, and making this a ritual will greatly increase your child's feelings of inner peace and joy.

### Step 1:
Take a notebook or exercise book and decorate it with pictures or drawings of things or people that you love.

### Step 2:
Write in it five things you are grateful for each day. This can be people, a situation that happened recently, a place, a pet or an object. Some days will be very similar, but try to vary it as much as you can.

Once you have established the practice of daily gratitude, you may want to add more than five. A tip is to write in your book at the same time each day; this will help you to form the habit. To establish the habit for your child, challenge them to do it for 30 days and have a calendar or timeline so that you can tick off each day.

YOU CAN change the world.
No matter what anyone says,
thoughts and ideas can change
the world. There is a lesson in
everything. Bad times always
wake you up to the stuff you
were not paying attention to.

——— Robin Williams ———

If you have enjoyed this book, please leave a review on Amazon. I'd love to know what you thought of it. I hope it can help you and your family.

For more advice on nutrition as well as an exclusive Nourish Your Teen recipe book, head over to my website:
**http://www.passionatenutrition.co.uk**

Printed in Great Britain
by Amazon